GO **Forward**

28 Days to Eat, Move,

and Enjoy Life God's Way

GO Forward

28 Days to Eat, Move,

and Enjoy Life God's Way

Sheri Traxler

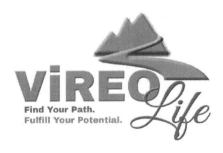

ISBN-13: 978-0692599914

ISBN-10: 0692599916

Every effort has been made to ensure that the information contained in the book is complete and accurate. However, the author is not engaged in rendering professional advice or services to the individual reader. The ideas, procedures, and suggestions contained in this book are not intended as a substitute for consulting with your physician. All matters regarding your health require medical supervision. The author shall not be liable or responsible for any loss, injury, or damage allegedly arising from any information or suggestion in this book.

To my mother,

Sarah Joann Edgington.

My mentor, friend, and first walking partner.

I look forward to walking with you again, on streets of
pure gold.

Acknowledgments

I am so grateful for all of you who have taught me the information and truths in this book. Thank you to the professors and professionals throughout my life who have patiently shared their knowledge with me, especially Jay Groves, Ph.D., Colin Armstrong, Ph.D., and all of the former and current staff of the Vanderbilt Dayani Center for Health and Wellness. Thank you to my clients and workshop participants, who teach me every day.

Thank you to my pastors who always speak truth without compromise. Thank you Pastor Maury Davis for your guidance, Pastor Sandy Sterban for your love and for editing the scripture usage in this book, and Pastor Bob Keich for your teaching and also editing this book's scripture usage.

My editor, Samantha Evilsizer, at Turned Editing Services – you are insightful and detailed. And thank you to all of my unofficial editors … Angie Spence, Jennifer McCoy, Patty Whitehead, Moren Adenubi, and the "small business Big God" Life Group members. You helped me communicate my passion. To my business and marketing team, Ron Doyle, Target One Coaching; Ron Hill, Clear Strategy Marketing; and Teri Lynne Underwood, you all keep me inspired and on track!

Thank you, more than I can articulate, to my favorite editor and best friend, Doug Traxler. Because of your patience, support, and encouragement, this book is going to change the lives of many people. You are my hero.

Finally, I have no words adequate to say THANK YOU to Jesus. Without Your sacrifice, I would have and be nothing. Thank You for your boundless love. God, You birthed in me as a child a desire to help people get healthy and You have guided my steps, through Your Holy Spirit, all of my life. I am so grateful for the opportunity to share Your Word about health through this book. May it, and my life, glorify You always.

Table of Contents

Dear Reader,

Please consult your physician before beginning an exercise program, or if you have health concerns requiring special attention.

I pray that the next 28 days will help you on your journey of health and inspire you to a closer relationship with God. If you are stuck on the diet-roller-coaster, or unmotivated to move, may the truth in the scriptures we will be studying set you free.

Best of health and life,

Sheri Traxler

The Day Before: How to Use this Guide

Your life is your journey. You have mountaintops you want to summit: your mission, dreams, and goals. God has given you a unique life to experience and live. By the very fact that it is *your* journey, you have to blaze your own trail. However, you don't have to walk without guidance. God will teach you the steps to take, just as He showed the Israelites their path to the Promised Land. In Joshua 3:4 God told the Israelites to follow the ark of the covenant, "that you may know the way by which you must go, for you have not passed this way before" (NKJV).

Whether you are beginning a healthy lifestyle for the first time (having "not passed this way before") or the fifth time, or overcoming a harmful habit, this devotional book will give you direction. It will help you move from goal to goal along your journey of health. It is a compass to help you find *your* path and fulfill *your* potential.

To use this book as your personal compass, I encourage you to study and practice Week One first. Week One's information will prepare you to succeed. Then review your goals, which you will be listing today. After Week One, you can read this book day-by-day or jump around to different days. Your steps could be any of the following:

- **Do you have a highest priority?** Study the section that guides you to that goal.
- **Do you enjoy challenges?** Look at your rockiest mountain and determine to climb it. Study the

1

section you find most difficult until you experience progress.
- **Do you need a quick win?** To give you momentum, start with a section – a path – that is easier for you.
- **Do you want to go step-by-step?** Journey straight through this devotional.

Ask the Holy Spirit to show you how you need to study and what you need to apply. He will help you and "accomplish what concerns" you (Psalm 138:8 NASB).

Each day is designed as follows:

- **Scripture:** read and reflect
- **My Thoughts:** consider what the scripture means to you. You can write your thoughts before and/or after you read the discussion.
- **Discussion:** learn about the topic
- **Your Challenge:** take action or ponder a thought to move you along your path
- **Scripture For Further Study:** look up verses for further reading. Sometimes these scriptures are about the "spiritual" side of a "practical" matter. For instance, many of the scriptures about water represent the Holy Spirit in you.

Please note that the Discussion section is not an exhaustive study of each topic. Devotions introduce an inspirational idea, help you to understand what the Bible says about that issue, and pique your hunger to study both Scripture and reputable health resources. As an example, on Day 10 we study strength training. That discussion teaches you what God's Word says about strength training and it encourages you to learn what types of strength training would be good for you. The appendix includes a resource for practical application.

Now that you understand how to follow along with this devotional, let's lace-up your walking shoes and begin your journey!

Here is your first challenge: Define some of your goals. (You can write them at the end of this introduction.)

Goals need to be specific. For example, if you want to eat more vegetables, how many servings do you want to average? If you desire to sleep more, how many hours of rest will you get each night? If you need to exercise more, how far will you walk each week? One important goal I encourage you to make is to read the Bible each day. Knowing God's Word will encourage you and give you the right perspective as you become healthier. To help you determine the details of your goals, choose both "outcome" goals and "behavior" goals.

An outcome goal is the result you want. **A behavior goal** is an action you take to achieve the result. For example, an outcome goal would be to lower your blood pressure to below 120/80. A behavior goal would be to walk three miles each day. You are in direct control of your behavior goals. You are not in direct control of your outcome goals, especially the exact timeframe in which you accomplish them. However, reaching for a challenging outcome makes changing behaviors more exciting!

Goals need to have a reason why. Think about the purpose of your goals. If you want to get stronger, ask yourself *why*? What are the benefits to your life once you are stronger? If you want to have more energy, ask yourself *why*? What are the benefits to your life once you are more energetic?

Your answers may vary: work without pain, set an example for your children, be physically able to play with your grandchildren, be alive to see your great-grandchildren, think more clearly at work, have energy at the end of the day to enjoy family time, or any other personal reasons. Think through your answers. When you have them, go ahead and record them here.

Your Challenge:

Write out your goals and why they are important to you:

_____

_____

_____

_____

_____

_____

_____

_____

_____

_____

Complete this commitment statement:

I am going to study God's Word each day at _____ o'clock.

Congratulations! You have set your goals. You've asked God to help you achieve those goals. You have prioritized time to invest in studying. The next step on your journey is to get a great night's sleep tonight (see *Day 22: From A(wake) to Zzz*). We are going to start finding *your* path tomorrow!

Week 1

Prepare to Succeed

Day 1: Is It God's Will ... or Is It Selfish?

Or do you not know that your body is a temple of the Holy Spirit who is in you, whom you have from God, and that you are not your own? For you have been bought with a price: therefore glorify God in your body. I Corinthians 6:19-20 (NASB)

For I do *not mean that others should be eased and you burdened.* 2 Corinthians 8:13 (NKJV)

Do nothing from selfishness or empty conceit, but with humility of mind regard one another as more important than yourselves; do not merely *look out for your own personal interests, but also for the interests of others.* Philippians 2:3-4 (NASB)

My Thoughts:

_____

_____

_____

Let's start with a concern you may have. "By taking time to exercise or relax or (fill in the blank), am I following God's will ... or am I being selfish?" This subconscious and nagging question often stops people from making lifestyle change. It is a cannot-win-trap for many of my

7

clients. If they do not take time to take care of themselves, they feel they are not being good stewards of the body God entrusted to them (1 Corinthians 6:19-20). If they do take time to take care of themselves, by doing something pleasurable and relaxing, they feel they are being selfish. They think they should spend that time working or serving others.

Let's address this concern by examining today's scriptures.

Your body is not your own. You were bought with a price and are a steward of your body, your time and your resources. God bought you with the sacrifice and blood of His Son, Jesus. Therefore, you are to glorify God and reflect Him in every area of your life, including the way you treat your body. Taking care of your temple helps you to be more productive and enjoy the life God gave you. According to 1 Timothy 6:17, enjoying your life is also God's will.

Your time and money are for both you and others. In a letter Paul wrote to the Galatians, he exhorts them to serve others, which includes giving their time (Galatians 5:13). He penned a separate letter to the local church in Corinth in which he encourages them to provide money to those in need in Jerusalem. However, in the middle of spurring the people to give monetarily, Paul shares a principle of balance in 2 Corinthians 8:13. I believe we can also apply this principle of balance to our time. Here is the principle: we should not give our money or our time to a point of burden for us, including defaulting on our debts, forgoing our responsibilities, or neglecting our health, so that others can have it easy.

Your balance is not selfish. Philippians 2:3-4 is a wonderfully balanced instruction that commands us not to be selfish. What is selfishness? According to the *Spirit Filled Life Bible* commentary, "selfish ambition" is a phrase that "regressed from denoting honorable work to suggesting dishonorable intrigue ... [it] later described a person who was concerned only with his own welfare, a person susceptible to being bribed, an ambitious, self-willed person seeking opportunities for promotion. From there it became electioneering, a partisan factious spirit that would resort to any method for winning followers."[i] Prioritizing time for a walk, cooking a healthy meal, or relaxing for an evening just somehow does not fall under the above description, does it?

Philippians 2:4 includes an important phrase: "Not merely … but also." What does that mean? If I said, "Our vacation was *not merely* fun, *but* it was *also* relaxing" then I am saying it was *both* fun *and* relaxing. Right? Philippians 2:4 includes looking out *both* for your own interests *and* for the interests of others. Since you are studying this devotional book, I assume your health is one of your own interests.

Your Challenge:

What steps will you take to look out *both* for your interests and for the interest of others?

_____

_____

_____

_____

_____

_____

_____

For Further Study: Galatians 6:2-5 and 1 Timothy 4:1

_____

_____

_____

_____

_____

_____

_____

_____

_____

_____

_____

_____

_____

_____

_____

_____

_____

_____

Day 2: Changing Habits

Meditate on these things; give yourself entirely to them, that your progress may be evident to all. 1 Timothy 4:15 (NKJV)

My Thoughts:

_____

_____

_____

You may have heard the saying, "It's lovely to know what to do; it's life-changing to do what you know." If you aren't doing what you know, today will help you begin the process. Changing your health habits, so that "your progress may be evident to all," requires two actions.

"Meditate on these things." In order to successfully move forward on your health journey, you will need to remove different obstacles. One hindrance is unhelpful thoughts such as, "I don't know if I can do this." Rather than thinking negative thoughts, meditate on what the Bible says, particularly in regard to your health.

Another hindrance is that we all live our current patterns by reflex and without thought. To change to a new manner of living, you must consciously choose your actions each moment, until the new way of living is automatic. How do you break an engrained pattern and start a new one? Think constantly on the new habit you want to form or the lifestyle you want to live. How do you keep your mind focused on a new habit? Use reminders and cues, such as the following:

- On your pantry door, post scriptures that inspire you to eat healthy
- Keep a pair of walking shoes at work
- Set your phone to ring when it is time to go workout
- Have a friend ask you about your new habit each week
- Join an online group that swaps healthy recipes

Since you will be changing strong habitual thought patterns and ways of living, you need to implement numerous reminders.

What reminders to "meditate on these things" will you put in place today?

Who can encourage you to think about your new health habit?

_____

_____

_____

_____

_____

"Give yourself entirely to them." Decrease or eliminate what distracts you from your goal. Do not have so many new goals that they distract from each other. Choose one or two new habits that reinforce each other to focus on at a time. For example: *I will drink two cups of water after my mid-day walk.* "Entirely" means one hundred percent. If you try to form several new healthy habits at once, you will not be able to give all of your attention to each. After a week (or a month) of practicing one habit, add another. What if you have a setback? No worries. Turn lapses into lessons. Do not judge yourself,

12

but learn from your experiences. This time next year the "new habits" will be a lifestyle.

On which one or two habits will you focus this week?

_____

_____

Your Challenge:

Begin confessing, "I determine the health habit on which I focus. With God's help, I meditate on it and do it. I surround myself with people who encourage me to live healthy." After a week of practice, evaluate if you need to change your reminders or add another habit.

_____

_____

_____

_____

_____

_____

_____

_____

For Further Study: 2 Corinthians 3:18 and Philippians 1:6

_____

_____

_____

_____

_____

_____

_____

_____

_____

_____

_____

_____

_____

_____

_____

_____

Day 3: Encourage Yourself

David was greatly distressed, for the men spoke of stoning him because the souls of them all were bitterly grieved, each man for his sons and daughters. But David encouraged and strengthened himself in the Lord his God.
1 Samuel 30:6 (AMP)

My Thoughts:

_____

_____

_____

What an amazing and challenging story! David and his men have just come back from battle; these warriors are exhausted and hungry (never a good combination). They are ready to see their families, yet arrive home to find their loved ones gone and their houses destroyed. David, in the middle of his own grief, also finds out his men are ready to kill him! In his trouble what does David do? Hide? Run away? No. He encourages himself in the Lord.

By God's grace, may we never face the level of distress that David and his men experienced. But from how David handled his trials we can glean a lesson for our own struggles.

As much as I wish it weren't so, I need to warn you that as you begin a new healthy lifestyle, there will be challenging days (sometimes weeks). Many factors can make choosing healthy habits difficult. People. Family. Work. Crises. Familiar habit triggers. Life. To help combat tough moments, it is critical that you know ahead of time what ...

- Encourages you
- Helps you to stick to your new habits
- Gets you back on track if you take a side step, which everyone does.

Encouragement is one of the most important lessons in these 28 days. Don't rush through today and tomorrow. If you need to stay here an extra few days, meditating on the scriptures and letting the Holy Spirit show you ideas of how to encourage yourself in the Lord, do it. Remember, this is your journey.

Your Challenge:

Make a list of what encourages you in other areas of life. How can you apply that list to sticking with your new habits?

For illustration, if listening to praise songs helps you, decide on a go-to song; when you recognize discouragement, start singing that song. If a particular book lifts you up, stash a copy at your desk and by your bed. If certain scriptures, quotes, or affirmations inspire you in tough times, write them on cards and keep them with you. You don't have to wait until discouragement attacks. You can sing and meditate now to stay ahead of the tough days.

Those are three simple examples. What are yours?

_____

_____

For Further Study: Judges 20:22 and Psalm 43:5

_____

_____

_____

_____

_____

_____

_____

_____

_____

_____

_____

_____

_____

_____

_____

_____

_____

_____

Day 4: Receive Encouragement

Two are better than one, because they have a good reward for their labor. For if they fall, one will lift up his companion. But woe to him who is alone when he falls, for he has no one to help him up. Ecclesiastes 4:9-10 (NKJV)

My Thoughts:

_____

_____

_____

Some days you encourage yourself in the Lord. Other days you need kind and uplifting encouragement from friends. Still other days you need an old-fashioned verbal toe kick, otherwise known as the "wounds of a friend." (Proverbs 27:6)

When it comes to picking friends who will help you to maintain your health habits, be choosy. Remember the ABC's of Friendship.

Select friends who:

- **Always encourage you** (Proverbs 12:25, Isaiah 50:4)
- **Believe in you** ("Is ever ready to the believe the best of every person." 1 Corinthians 13:7, AMP)

18

- **Correct and sharpen you** ("As iron sharpens iron." Proverbs 27:17, NKJV)
- **Don't tell others about your mistakes** ("Love covers all sins." Proverbs 10:12, NKJV)

How can a friend help you? Some individuals need a friend with whom they meet at the park to walk, go to the farmers market, or swap recipes. One of my clients prefers to exercise alone, but has asked a friend, "Can I message you when I don't feel like exercising?" Accountability and encouragement in some form are critical.

Your Challenge:

Ask God to show *who* can help you and *how* they can help you; list their names and your ideas below. He designed us to need each other.

Ask them if they are willing. If they say no, think of someone else.

1. _____

_____

2. _____

_____

3. _____

_____

4. _____

_____

5. _____

   _____

Now, let's take it another step. Sow a seed of
encouragement that will come back to you. Stop and ask
God, "Who needs reminding that they will make it and that
they will succeed?" Then sow the ABC's of Friendship
today. When you need it, you'll reap the encouragement
you've sown.

For Further Study: 1 Samuel 23:16, Proverbs 13:20, Proverbs 27:6, Isaiah 35:3, and 1 Thessalonians 5:11

_____

_____

_____

_____

_____

_____

_____

_____

_____

_____

_____

_____

_____

_____

_____

_____

Day 5: Get Help

Where there is no guidance the people fall, But in abundance of counselors there is victory. Proverbs 11:14 (NASB)

My Thoughts:

_____

_____

_____

I grew up reading Nancy Drew books. (Confession: I still read them.) Nancy knows about everything; she is an expert sailor, horse rider, golfer, dancer, skier, artist and award-winning floral designer. She is the person to whom everyone looks for answers, and she always solves the mystery. I would love to be that knowledgeable and an expert in everything, but that is not realistic. It is not even possible. It is fiction.

Therefore, in my real life, I need specialized experts to share their knowledge and skills with me. I need an "abundance of counselors." So do you.

Let's discover what counselors you need. Take your time answering these questions and come back to them in a couple of days, as new ideas will surface.

What are your top two health and wellness goals?

_____

_____

_____

What are your barriers to reaching those goals?

_____

_____

_____

What information, skills or support do you need to overcome those barriers?

_____

_____

_____

Who can provide that information or support to you?

Doctor/PCP

_____

Personal Trainer

_____

Nutrition Specialist or Registered Dietician

_____

Health Coach
_____

Books or Audio Recordings
_____

Workshops
_____

Other
_____

A friend of mine epitomizes overcoming barriers. He lost two limbs in an unusual and life-altering accident. I want to share with you the wisdom he uses to conquer obstacles. He knows that to fulfill his potential and to live his God-given dreams, he must:

- Be as healthy as possible (*Days Nine* through *Eleven: Get Fit*)
- Maintain supportive relationships (*Day Four: Receive Encouragement* and *Day 26: Relationships*)
- (Today's topic) *Get Help* for uncommonly creative exercise routines.

Hopefully, you do not have an extreme physical situation or daunting difficulties to hurdle. Whatever your barriers, remember you do not have to overcome them alone. There are experts to guide you.

Your Challenge:

This week, contact at least one group or person who can counsel you.

For Further Study: Proverbs 12:15, Proverbs 13:20, Proverbs 15:22, and Proverbs 24:6

_____

_____

_____

_____

_____

_____

_____

_____

_____

_____

_____

_____

_____

_____

_____

_____

Day 6: Who Is in Control?

But the fruit of the Spirit is love, joy, peace, longsuffering, kindness, goodness, faithfulness, gentleness, self-control. Against such there is no law.
Galatians 5:22-23 (NKJV)

My Thoughts:

_____

_____

_____

What controls your life? Generally, there are three options.

1. Rules and the endless "should's" about what you eat or how you exercise. These have false guilt associated with them.
2. The mood and feeling of the moment with no thought of future impact.
3. Self-control.

Let's take a brief look at the first two options, and then we'll discuss the last one.

First, *external* control (rules and regulations) will not work for nourishing or moving your body. In *Day 15: Why Don't Diets Work?* we will study Colossians 2:20-23, which teaches us the truth about *external* control.

Second, *no* control is also not God's way. Study Galatians 5, Ephesians 3, and Colossians 3 for a glimpse of what God says about *no* control.

Third, the good news is that you have something better than external or no control. As a Christian, you are a new creation in Christ with a new nature that never existed before your salvation (2 Corinthians 5:17). Included in your new nature is *self*-control. Do you have an old flesh man with old habits, including no control, which you must crucify? Yes. Do you have a mind and thinking patterns you must renew? Yes. You also have a new man inside you that actually *wants and enjoys* doing what is beneficial. *Self*-control trains the new man to get louder and the old man to hush up.

How do you strengthen your self-control? Here are two ideas.

1. **Positive Reinforcement**. Each time you use self-control ("I *choose* to eat my veggies because I feel better when I do") instead of external rules ("I *have to have* broccoli tonight because ..."), congratulate yourself.

   Each time you use self-control instead of no control, reward yourself. For example, when you think, "I know I'd have more energy if I walked, but this sofa is so comfortable," but you get up and walk *anyway.*

2. **Practice Knowledge.** Second Peter 1:6, in the Amplified Bible, tells us that "exercising knowledge" develops self-control. Educate yourself on the hundreds of benefits of exercise, nutritious foods, intuitive eating and healthy living. It is easier to eat your broccoli and go for a walk when you know all of the ways these renew your body.

Once you get some knowledge on the benefits and how-to's of healthy living, *practice* it. Be aware: when you begin something new, it does not feel natural. Expect new thoughts and actions to feel foreign to you. Practice anyway. You will not do it very well at first and will likely stumble. That is normal. Pick yourself up and go forward anyway.

Do not wait until you have researched all aspects of a health habit before you try what you have learned. It is impossible to learn all the knowledge you need in one moment. Philippians 3:16 says, "Only let us hold true to what we have already attained *and* walk *and* order our lives by that." (AMP) Attain some knowledge. Practice it. Attain more knowledge. Practice it.

Your Challenge:

Begin confessing, "I control myself today. External rules do not control me. I obey the voice of my new man inside me." Ask God to show you where you need *self*-control and then *practice it.*

For Further Study: Proverbs 12:24, Romans 8:2, 1 Corinthians 9:25, Galatians 5, Ephesians 3, and Colossians 3

_____

_____

_____

_____

_____

_____

_____

_____

_____

_____

_____

_____

_____

_____

_____

_____

Day 7: You're Worth It!

She makes tapestry for herself, her clothing is fine linen and purple. Proverbs 31:22 (NKJV)

My Thoughts:

_____

_____

_____

The woman described in Proverbs 31 managed a full household, ran at least two successful businesses, ministered to the poor, and lived in a way that her family loved and respected her. When men and women read Proverbs 31, they are frequently overwhelmed and wonder, "How does she do it all?" There are many principles within the passage that offer answers, but those are for another book. For now, let's focus on one precept: the treasure in verse 22.

While this woman managed, worked, and gave, she also took time to take care of herself. For example, compare what she sold with what she wore. She made *linen* sashes to sell. But she wore *fine* linen and *purple* clothing. (Study Proverbs 31:22 and 31:24 in various translations.)

Colorful clothes from fine linen may not seem like a big deal now, but a few thousand years ago, you would read that and say, "Seriously? Wow!" Then you'd post it on all of your social media accounts! You see, laborers used sea snails to make purple dye. It took about 12,000 of those smelly creatures to accumulate 1.4 grams of purple dye. The historian Theopompus wrote "Purple for dyes fetched its weight in silver." That was the stuff royalty could afford. Ponder this: the Proverbs 31 woman owned *at least* one set of purple clothing.

My brush with that kind of luxury happened a few years ago during a trip to Chicago. While there, I decided to visit the Chanel boutique. I knew it couldn't hurt to try something on, so I did: three beautiful Chanel jackets, worth about $5,000 each. I thought to myself, "I just tried on a new car in five minutes. Wow." I now joke in workshops, when I'm teaching the principle of self-care, that yes, the Proverbs 31 woman did serve and work hard … and she did it all in a Chanel suit.

Beyond caring for herself with the clothes she wore, the woman in Proverbs 31 also made tapestry for herself. She prioritized time to create something that she wanted.

The New Testament also encourages this balanced way of living. On *Day One: Is It God's Will … or is It Selfish?*, we studied Philippians 2:4, "Let each of you look out not only for his own interests, but also for the interests of others" (NKJV). This verse presupposes you are taking care of your own interests. The woman of Proverbs 31 is a clear illustration of how to live balanced. She did not think, "It's all about me," but neither did she neglect her needs.

Many clients tell me, "I want to take care of both myself and others, but there is not enough time or money." If you feel this same way, be encouraged! It is possible for you to do both. How? By changing the way you invest your time and money, using one of two methods. Implement whichever one is best for you, or use a combination of both.

Method One: OUT-IN

Take OUT of your life what does not bring good
results so that you have room to bring IN what does. For
the OUT-IN method, it is important to answer a few
questions about your time and your money:

- What current responsibilities are God-ordained?
  What ones are not?
- What current activities do not improve your health,
  relax you, build your relationships, or move you
  closer to your goals? In other words, where is
  your time not invested well?
- What is your current budget? What do you spend
  money on that does not satisfy you in the long-
  term?

Once you have your answers, begin to eliminate OUT
self-inflicted responsibilities, low-impact activities, and
frivolous spending. This opens up time and money in your
life to care for yourself.

Method Two: IN-OUT

Define clear and exact results you desire in your
health and your life. Every day bring IN only actions and
choices that align with your goals. This moves you closer
to your desired outcomes, and it automatically takes OUT
waste of your scheduling and spending.

Whichever method you choose, do not wait until you
have all of the time and money you think you need. You
can practice self-care now. You don't have to spend
money on a luxury suit or make tapestries for yourself. (I
personally have no interest in weaving.) Start with
something small and inexpensive. Aim to be like the
woman in Proverbs 31 and stay within your household
budget. (Read Proverbs 31:12. "Does him good" includes
not going into debt buying that fine linen purple robe.)
Use your imagination: walk at the mall instead of the gym,

grow a backyard garden or find a farmers market, hunt for exercise equipment at yard sales, watch free online exercise videos, or trade kid-care nights with a friend to open time in your schedule to relax.

Your Challenge:

Make a list of at least 10 ways you can take care of yourself that you are not currently doing. Decide which one or two you can implement within the next two weeks and do them. If there is something on the list which you cannot afford right now, whether hiring a certified trainer or going to a spa, begin saving for it. You are worth it!

_____

_____

_____

_____

_____

_____

_____

For Further Study: Genesis 1:31, Psalm 37:3-5, and
Psalm 139:14-15

Week 2

What Does the Bible Say

about Exercise?

Day 8: Is Exercise Essential to Godly Living?

For bodily exercise profits a little, but godliness is profitable for all things, having promise of the life that now is and of that which is to come. 1 Timothy 4:8 (NKJV)

Who can find a virtuous wife? For her worth is far above rubies. Proverbs 31:10 (NKJV)

She girds herself with strength [spiritual, mental, and physical fitness for her God-given task] and makes her arms strong and firm. Proverbs 31:17 (AMP)

My Thoughts:

_____

_____

_____

Hmmm. So is the Holy Spirit, through Paul, saying exercise is not important? Once we examine these scriptures and history, you will be able to answer that question.

According to 1 Timothy 4:8, bodily exercise is profitable, though *not as much as* training for godliness. In Proverbs chapter 31, verses 10 and 17 together teach that physical exercise is *part of* godliness. How can exercise both be *part of* godliness and be *less beneficial than* godliness? To reconcile these two ideas, we must understand "exercise" as Paul's readers did 2000 years ago.

Athletes practiced for the Olympic Games, which were held from 776 B.C. to 393 A.D. Roman Gladiators also physically trained for their deadly competitions. In 1 Timothy 4:8, we see that the Greek word "gumnasia" is translated "exercise" or "training." Its root word, "gumnazo," means training "for the games." Athletic events were so central to Greek culture, metaphorically and physically, most cities had a gymnasium at their center. Paul's travels would have made him familiar with athletes disciplining their bodies for competition. His readers would have understood the imagery he used in his writings and called it "exercise."

We have similar training today. If you have watched a Strongman Competition, our modern-day Olympics, or a local swim meet, you have seen the profitable outcomes of the athletes' hard work. However, we don't usually equate their extraordinary workouts with simple "exercise;" we call it "athletic training."

As another comparison, physical labor comprised a major component of life in biblical times. Everyday activities required and built stamina. If you lived in Paul's day, you would have regularly walked from Bethany to Jerusalem and back to Bethany. You'd have logged about four miles roundtrip (John 11:18) and simply said, "I went to town." When you walk four miles today, what do you say? "I exercised."

We have established two ideas:

1. We differ from Paul's contemporaries in our definition of "exercise."
2. Paul is comparing "athletic training" (not "exercise") with training for godliness.

With this history under our belt, we can now answer today's title question, "Is exercise essential to godly living?" Yes. Allow me to explain.

Proverbs 31 gives us a picture of a virtuous, excellent, godly woman who kept her body fit for her tasks. If you recall from *Day Seven: You're Worth It!*, that includes looking out for her interests, as well as the interests of others. How does this translate to you and me, and what does it have to do with godliness?

Regular physical activity enables us to manage our homes, run our businesses, take care of ourselves, and minister to others. Being physically fit allows us to mow our yards, keep up with our kids, clean an elderly friend's home, or serve at a soup kitchen. Doing our best to stay healthy allows us to glorify God fully, for all of our lives. Exercise *is* essential to godly living.

Your Challenge:

Begin confessing, "I profit in all things. I strive for godliness, including physical well-being."

Day 9: Get Fit Part One – Cardiovascular

Endurance

She girds herself with strength [spiritual, mental, and physical fitness for her God-given task] and makes her arms strong and firm. Proverbs 31:17 (AMP)

My Thoughts:

_____

_____

_____

Over the next three days we will focus on three aspects of physical fitness:

- Cardiovascular endurance
- Strength
- Flexibility

Today's focus is on increasing your cardiovascular health and fitness for your "God-given tasks." Think about the tasks God has assigned to you in your *current* season of life. Visualize your days and your weeks.

List your regular tasks (be as detailed as possible).

_____

_____

_____

What do you need from your spirit, mind, and body to perform those tasks? For example, do you need more _mental sharpness_ at work? Do you want _energy_ when you get home to re-paint a room, or _endurance_ to play sports with your kids? **Write what you need below.**

_____

_____

_____

Now think about your tasks for your _next_ season of life. Do you look forward to keeping up with your grandchildren (and great-grandchildren) at a theme park? Will you want to live independently, even making minor home repairs, throughout your life? Do you want to _decrease your risk of major diseases_ so you are alive at 100 years of age to still fulfill your calling? (Moses had 20 years to go at that point!) **List your _next_ season tasks here.**

_____

_____

_____

To enjoy the benefits you have listed above, invest a little time each day _now_ to strengthen your heart. Move your body. How?

41

There are three options to mix and match, depending on your schedule.

1. **Solo shot:** Schedule one stretch of time for exercise. For example, go for a three mile walk after dinner each evening.
2. **Short shots:** Perhaps your schedule does not allow for a 45-60 minute block. Solution? Take three separate 15-minute walks: one before work, one at lunch and one in the evening.
3. **Step shots:** Invest in an accurate pedometer or GPS (satellite) driven fitness tracker. (Note that some GPS controlled fitness trackers do not accurately measure steps on a treadmill.) Then find your average daily number of steps and add approximately 6,000 steps to the baseline. This combined number is now your daily step goal. You can also shoot for 10,000 steps per day. Build up slowly and creatively. You could walk at the park while your son's soccer team is warming up or walk in place during commercials.

These are ideas for helping you begin to incorporate physical activity to improve your cardiovascular endurance. (A certified personal trainer will be able to help you design a specific program for your goals.)

God calls the person who is physically active "capable, intelligent, and virtuous" (Proverbs 31:10, AMP). Remember, it is not just about being able to climb a mountain when you are 120 years old, like Moses. Numerous studies show a significant link between physical exercise and mental sharpness and emotional health. To stay strong mentally, emotionally, and physically ... stop sitting and start moving.

(If you have health concerns, get your doctor's clearance and professional advice before increasing your exercise. Do not wait.)

Your Challenge:

Begin confessing, "Every day I find ways to move the only body God gave to me." Decide *how* you will experiment with the three cardiovascular fitness options this week or *whom* you need to contact for clearance to exercise.
Then do it.

Day 10: Get Fit Part Two – Strength Training

> She *girds herself with strength [spiritual, mental, and physical fitness for her God-given task] and makes her arms strong and firm.* Proverbs 31:17 (AMP)

My Thoughts:

_____

_____

_____

Yesterday we discussed cardiovascular endurance. Let's go to the next level of physical fitness, which is muscular strength. If we read "makes her arms strong and firm" as a literal statement, the woman in Proverbs 31 did some version of strength training.

Stop for a moment and look back at your lists from yesterday. Today's study will be much more effective with your lists fresh on your mind.

Now, think about which tasks require not just cardiovascular health and endurance, but also muscular strength. Do you want to try a new activity – whether gardening, kayaking, fly-fishing, or _____ – without pain? Do you want to go on a mission trip to help repair homes or build churches? Do you want to lift your own grocery bags when you are 90 years old?

While I won't suggest a particular strength training program, as everyone is vastly different in his or her

44

needs, I will say it doesn't take as much time as most people think for general improvements. Twenty to thirty minutes, two to three days per week, is all it takes for a basic strength program. Of course, your goals may require a bit more time.

A typical program might include lifting free weights, doing pliés at a ballet barre, using resistance bands, working out on weight machines, or a combination of these exercises. There are several great videos, programs and books on strength training

Here are some tips for evaluating them for your use:

1. Does the program show options for beginner, intermediate, and advanced levels?
2. Are there demonstrations and explanations you can understand for safety?
3. Does the program include modifications for various "joint issues," especially knee, lower back, and shoulders? (For example, if you have knee problems, you may need to modify your range of motion, when doing squats.)
4. Are all of the major muscle groups (legs, chest, back) emphasized?
5. Are the minor muscle groups (arms, shoulders, calves) and abdomen included?
6. Does the program describe safety tips, such as lifting speed, breathing, partner training, and rest time between exercises?
7. Is there a variety of exercises from which to choose?

If you are training with strength machines at a gym, ask a certified personal trainer to show you how to adjust each machine for your height. Machines can be very safe, but alignment is critical for the health of your joints.

General safety tips:

1. **Recuperate:** Give your muscle fibers a minimum of 48 hours to heal. If you train your chest muscles on Monday, then Wednesday would be the earliest you would train them again.
2. **Rotate:** Rotate each week between different exercises for the same muscles. It is not only more interesting, but it helps to prevent overuse injury to your joints.
3. **Rest:** If something twinges, do not override your body's signal. Let it rest for a few minutes or even a few days, before you exercise that muscle group again. If the twinge continues, talk with a certified personal trainer, physical therapist, or your healthcare provider to evaluate next steps.
4. **Re-assess:** If something moves from twinging to hurting, stop. Then get with a professional for advice.

God wants you to be strong. A few of the scriptures concerning physical strength are included For Further Study. Read over these, and use them as inspiration to begin, or continue, your strength training regime.

Your Challenge:

Research resources, classes and/or trainers to begin your strength training routine. If you are already on a regular program, pat yourself on the back! Good job!

For Further Study: Genesis 49:24, Joshua 14:11, 1
Chronicles 26:8, Nehemiah 4:10, Psalm 18:39, Psalm
33:16, Isaiah 40:29-31, Mark 12:30-33, and Acts 14:8-10

_____

_____

_____

_____

_____

_____

_____

_____

_____

_____

_____

_____

_____

_____

_____

_____

Day 11: Get Fit Part Three – Flexibility

She girds herself with strength [spiritual, mental, and physical fitness for her God-given task] and makes her arms strong and firm. Proverbs 31:17 (AMP)

My Thoughts:

_____

_____

_____

I searched for a scripture specific to flexibility, our final physical fitness topic. I found none, except to take a portion of Proverbs 31:19 completely out of context: "She stretches." (I know. Poor attempt at humor.) Since I'm not going to push the boundaries of Scripture, let's continue with the principle taught in Proverbs 31:17: you are to make your body able to work and serve.

You can be extremely strong and extremely *in*flexible. I see it in gyms constantly. *In*flexibility keeps athletes from reaching their potential, and it keeps individuals from fully enjoying life. How? What does flexibility do for you?

Flexibility:

1. Decreases risk and severity of injury
2. Increases mobility for general daily activity
3. Increases sports performance

48

4. Improves posture (lower back pain, anyone?)
5. Improves coordination

If these benefits sound appealing, you might be asking yourself how to attain them. How do you improve your flexibility? Simple. Stretch. Lengthening your muscles takes only a few minutes each day and requires no equipment. Stretching not only increases your flexibility, but it improves blood supply to your joints, which means nutrients are brought in and waste is removed.

Stretching tips:

1. **How often should you stretch?** To increase your flexibility, stretch every day.
2. **When should you stretch?** Anytime. However, you will gain the most flexibility for your effort when you stretch after a workout.
3. **How far should you stretch?** If you stretch right after you wake up, remember that your muscles are not "warmed up," so keep stretches gentle. You should barely be able to feel a stretch. If you stretch after exercising, you can push a little farther, but never to a point of pain.
4. **How long should you hold a stretch?** Hold your stretches for five to 60 seconds. Length of time will depend on your flexibility goals, previous injuries, or how often during the day you stretch.
5. **Where should you stretch?** Some stretching is always better than none. Don't allow limited time or different locations to deter you. You may not start with a 10-minute stretching routine at home or the gym, but you can do a few stretches while waiting in line, waiting for an appointment, standing at the copier (I've gotten a few laughs from coworkers while stretching in the copy room, but it keeps me flexible), talking on the phone, or watching TV.

Your Challenge:

Start stretching for a few minutes each day, especially after walking or another exercise.

Day 12: Be Safe

The plans of the diligent lead surely to plenty, but those of everyone who is hasty, surely to poverty. Proverbs 21:5 (NKJV)

A faithful man will abound with blessings, but he who makes haste to be rich will not go unpunished. Proverbs 28:20 (NASB)

My Thoughts:

_____

_____

_____

After reading today's scripture, you may be wondering, "What does exercise have to do with being rich?" A lot. In a survey of 50 billionaires, 80% exercise regularly. Fifty percent workout at least five days each week, and another 29% exercise two to three days per week.[ii] (Perhaps you want to go back to the outcome goals you initially listed and add "increase my net worth.") The connection between health and wealth is for another book though.

For today, let's look at another principle we can extrapolate from today's scripture: when you are diligent over time, you will be rewarded; when you rush in an area, you will suffer unwanted consequences. Whether dealing with money or starting a new exercise routine, be wise and be safe. Do not be hasty. Don't get me wrong, I rejoice with your excitement and determination to start exercising! Celebrate your resolve. Take deliberate action. Just *be safe*.

We've all heard the "success stories" about runners finishing marathons or individuals losing 50 pounds through high-intensity training. Not realizing that those achievements started with something less intense, people find the stories inspiring, get excited (good), and jump into a 45-minute interval class with both dusty sneakers (not good). They go for a two mile run with sprints and come home with throbbing knees and aching ankles. Of course, that means a few days of pain and recovery. Their enthusiasm wears off, and it is another year before they try it again.

Rather than diving into the deep end, one effective method is to "start slow." I hear you thinking, "Yeah, all right. That's not helpful. What does slow even mean?" (I understand your frustration. When my husband and I started gardening, we knew nothing, including how much to plant. Experienced gardeners warned us, "Start slow. Don't plant an area larger than you can keep weeded." Unfortunately that advice was not specific enough since, as novice gardeners, we had no idea how fast weeds grew! But that's another story.)

"Start slow" for exercise means to increase pace or time by no more than 10% each week. Let's take walking as an example.

Test how long you can walk at a moderate pace, at which you are able to carry on a conversation, before you feel your legs or lungs beginning to work, but not hurt. What length of time did you record? Five minutes? Twenty minutes? Thirty minutes? That is your starting point for Week One (and additional weeks, if needed). Increase either your pace *or* time by no more than 10% per week.

For example, perhaps 20 minutes for one mile is your starting point, and you plan to walk 20 minutes at lunch each day.

- Week One: 20 minutes, 1 mile
- Week Two: 20 minutes, 1.1 miles
- Week Three: 20 minutes, 1.2 miles

Perhaps you plan to walk every evening, and you want to keep the same pace, but increase your time each week.

- Week One: 20 minutes, 1 mile
- Week Two: 22 minutes, 1.1 miles
- Week Three: 24 minutes, 1.2 miles

Hopefully that gives you an idea of what "don't be hasty" with your exercise means. You can also apply the 10% guideline to your strength and flexibility routines.

There are numerous factors in designing a safe exercise program, beyond the scope of this devotional guide. I encourage you to get with a certified personal trainer or exercise physiologist to design a program specific to your goals and lifestyle.

Of course all of this assumes you have no health issues which need to be discussed with your doctor prior to exercise. If you have health issues, please let your doctor know that you plan to begin an exercise program: he/she can decide your next step, based on your last physical. If you don't have a doctor, or if you haven't had a physical in the past year, get one. Period.

Your Challenge:

If you are not currently on a regular exercise program, decide your starting point – whether a daily walk or a call to your doctor – and take action on it.

For Further Study: Proverbs 28:22

_____

_____

_____

_____

_____

_____

_____

_____

_____

_____

_____

_____

_____

_____

_____

_____

_____

_____

_____

Day 13: Extreme Fitness

Then Jesus went out from there [Gennesaret, see Matthew 14:34] *and departed to the region of Tyre and Sidon.* Matthew 15:21 (NKJV)

Jesus departed from there [Tyre and Sidon], *skirted the Sea of Galilee, and went up on the mountain and sat down there.* Matthew 15:29 (NKJV)

My Thoughts:

_____

_____

_____

If 2000 years ago I started a television program called *Extreme Fitness: 30 A.D.*, I would feature Jesus on the show. This idea is not to dishonor our Lord. I am simply amazed at His conditioning.

To better understand the fitness level of Jesus, explore His journeys. For today's study, find a map of Palestine during the time of Christ, in the back of your Bible or on the Internet. Follow along Jesus' route in Matthew 15:21 and 29.

Let's pick up the story in Matthew 15:21. We find Jesus teaching in Gennesaret, which is located near the northwest corner of the Sea of Galilee. He leaves Gennesaret and travels northward to Tyre and Sidon. Between these two regions wind 35-50 rough mountainous miles. Jesus either covers the distance in a day, or He sleeps outside overnight, likely in the mountains. Either option is physically demanding. After healing a Canaanite woman's daughter in the area of Tyre and Sidon, He turns around and walks back over the mountains to the Sea of Galilee, this time skirting the sea on the east side through the region of Decapolis (Mark 7:31).

Reading Matthew 15:29, I laughed to myself. "If I had just hiked from Gennesaret to Tyre and Sidon, then back to and around the Sea of Galilee, I would be sore and I would sit down, too!" However, that is not why Jesus sat down. The practice of that time was for teachers to be seated. In fact, Jesus still had enough physical stamina for the anointing to flow through Him. Read the next verse. Matthew 15:30 says, "Then great multitudes came to Him, having with them *the* lame, blind, mute, maimed, and many others; and they laid them down at Jesus' feet, and He healed them" (NKJV). Stop and think about that. Remember, He had the same physical limitations as you and I. In addition, Jesus worked as a carpenter; this was a very physical profession, especially with the use of only hand tools.

I don't believe God asks us to hike 70-100 strenuous miles in order to be healthy. However, I do believe He wants us to exercise regularly, maybe even a specific amount. I am not called to a physically demanding job; perhaps you aren't either, though many are. Either way, we can apply Proverbs 31:17 and make sure that we stay strong enough to fulfill our calling throughout our entire lives.

How is God asking you to exercise? God created your body and knows what it needs. Ask Him to show you the amount of time, pace, and types of exercise that will most benefit your body for His glory.

Your Challenge:

Spend time in prayer today asking God to show you what exercise to incorporate into your life.

For Further Study: Matthew 15:21-39 and Mark 7:24-8:10; note that the 70-100 mile roundtrip includes one recorded miracle: healing a Gentile woman's daughter.

_____

_____

_____

_____

_____

_____

_____

_____

_____

_____

_____

_____

_____

_____

_____

Day 14: Be in Health

Beloved, I pray that in all respects you may prosper and be in good health, just as your soul prospers. 3 John 2 (NASB)

My Thoughts:

_____

_____

_____

Describe what the phrase "be in good health" means to you.

_____

_____

_____

While we know what good health looks and feels like, the concept can be difficult to describe. According to the World Health Organization (WHO), "Health is a state of complete physical, mental and social well-being and not merely the absence of disease or infirmity."[iii] In addition to WHO's definition, I like the view that health is the capacity to overcome challenges.

One elucidating image of wellness is a continuum. Picture a line with disease on one end and complete, or perfect, well-being on the other. Everyone's level of wellness is somewhere on that line.

Disease ◀----------------------▶ Health

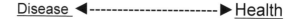

Health is not "either/or" or "all or nothing." When dealing with a physical issue, seeing health on a continuum is a hope-filled perspective. An injury or illness does not mean the end of health. Though you may be limited in your physical abilities, there is most likely some form of exercise you can perform. For example, "I may have a knee problem, but I can swim to keep my heart healthy." The same is true if you have a sickness or a disease. "Until my healing manifests, I'm managing _____, but I can still work and play." You can focus on the positive as you progressively improve your health overall.

(Just a quick warning to those with perfectionist tendencies: the continuum concept can be frustrating because there is no end-point. Since you will always be able to improve in an area of fitness or health, you will never be able to say, "I am 100% as fit and healthy as possible in every area." Relax. Define health as your ability to adapt, while moving toward greater health each day by God's grace. Know that you'll be "as fit and healthy as possible" in your resurrected body.)

My personal definition has evolved over the years. For me health is possessing the abundant energy and ability necessary to fulfill God's calling, both today *and in light of the future*. For example, individuals who neglect relationships may not have emotional support when troubles come. Or, individuals who smoke are damaging their lungs. Maybe the damage is slight enough today that they can still do their work and enjoy their life, but the damage will compound and hurt their ability later in life.

Look back at your description of "be in good health." It likely includes some of the following:

Alert and energetic

Beneficial relationships

Enjoy life and a sense of well-being

Excellent posture

Few/no aches and pains

Good bone density

Good digestion

Happy

High self-confidence

Normal blood pressure

Normal cholesterol and triglycerides

Normal weight

Organs and systems functioning well

Peaceful mind, managing stressors

Physical endurance

Prevent various diseases

Strong and flexible muscular system

Strong immune system

Guess what? Studies consistently show that exercise helps you achieve all of those health benefits and many, many more!

Your Challenge:

What benefits of exercise encourage you the most? Think about them as you are exercising this week. Write your personal definition of health.

_____

_____

_____

_____

_____

For Further Study: Genesis 43:28, Proverbs 3:8, and
Proverbs 4:22

_____

_____

_____

_____

_____

_____

_____

_____

_____

_____

_____

_____

_____

_____

_____

_____

Week 3

What Does the Bible Say about Nutrition?

Day 15: Why Don't Diets Work?

So let no one judge you in food or in drink, or regarding a festival or a new moon or sabbaths …Therefore, if you died with Christ from the basic principles of the world, why, as though living in the world, do you subject yourselves to regulations – 'Do not touch, do not taste, do not handle,' … These things indeed have an appearance of wisdom in self-imposed religion, false humility, and neglect of the body, but are of no value against the indulgence of the flesh. Colossians 2:16, 20, 21, 23 (NKJV)

My Thoughts:

_____

_____

_____

Does the Bible promote dieting? No. At least not in the way our modern world defines dieting. "You mean I can eat tons of junk food everyday?" No, not that either (but we'll get to that when we talk about nutrition and stewardship of your body).

For now, it's important to understand that the world teaches you to follow an external set of regulations in terms of what you eat – *a diet*. Depending on what new book or fad is being promoted, that set of regulations changes every month. Here's the bottom line on diets: they don't work.

While science and research continually update sound nutritional knowledge, the spin-off fads and extremes only cause confusion. That is a clue that diets are not of God because 1 Corinthians 14:33 teaches us that "God is not the author of confusion" (NKJV). If diets are not of God, then the likelihood of them working long-term is slim (pun intended).

Have you ever followed a rigid plan of "eat only this" and "don't eat that" just to overeat every food you've banned? Have you *limited* the time of day you ate, *restricted* yourself to certain combinations of foods, or *counted* calories, only to constantly think about food? Did you then start eating when you weren't even hungry?

Those "regulations" obviously are of "no value against the indulgence of the flesh." In fact, Romans 7:4-6 says that those external regulations can actually stimulate the flesh. This is *one* reason why diets don't work. (There are actually numerous physiological and psychological reasons, which you can study in the resources listed in the appendix.)

God does not leave you without guidance, however. He provides wisdom in how to nourish your body. We will discover that over the next few days.

A next-to-final thought: The type of dieting I have discussed today relates to weight loss, not restrictions for a medical condition. If you are on a medical diet for a medical reason, please continue following the guidelines of your healthcare provider. Follow the principle of Proverbs 12:15: listen to wise counsel.

A final thought: dieting can lead to eating disorders. If you think you may have an eating disorder or have a concern about someone who may, please seek help from a mental health professional. Resources are listed in the appendix.

Your Challenge:

Begin confessing "I no longer look to external regulations. I will seek the Father, not the world's laws, for wisdom in my eating."

For Further Study: Romans 7:4-12

_____

_____

_____

_____

_____

_____

_____

_____

_____

_____

_____

_____

_____

_____

_____

_____

Day 16: It's a Good Thing

Who satisfies your mouth with good things, so that your youth is renewed like the eagle's. Psalm 103:5 (NKJV)

My Thoughts:

_____

_____

_____

Take a moment to answer the following questions before reading further.

1. Who is the "Who" in the verse above?

    _____

2. What signals does your body give 20 minutes to two hours after eating that a food is a "good thing"–or is not a "good thing?"

    _____

3. What signals does your body give over weeks/months that a food is a "good thing"–or is not a "good thing?"

    _____

4. Describe what renewing "your youth" means in your life.

_____

_____

_____

There are many applications for this scripture. Let's see how it relates to nutrition.

First, God made your body. He created the foods that your body knows best how to use versus man's overly-processed foods your body often rejects (with stomachaches, headaches, joint pains, weight gain, etc.).

Second, the Hebrew word for "renew" is "chadash," which means to "rebuild and repair." Therefore, a food is a "good thing" if it rebuilds and repairs your body. As an obvious example, an apple will rebuild your body's cells more than an apple turnover. That does not mean you cannot have an apple turnover, pasta carbonara, or your favorite _____. Recall yesterday's lesson on setting up "external regulations" and why diets don't work.

Your Challenge:

Today's challenge is quite intensive. Begin confessing, "I commit to eating a variety of foods, close to how God made them, so that my health and energy ('my youth') is rebuilt."

1. List foods that you often eat which either:

- Don't satisfy you or give you sustained energy, but leave you feeling bloated, shaky, or moody.
- Your physician or registered dietician have told you are not healthy for your body right now.

_____

_____

Now, list alternative foods you enjoy and find satisfying.

_____

_____

2. List your 10 favorite "good things … renew your youth" foods.

_____

_____

_____

_____

_____

_____

3. Swap out recipes. Get out your cookbooks or search on the Internet for 10 (yes, 10) meal ideas which incorporate your alternatives and/or favorite "good things" foods.

4. Prepare. Plan how to add these meals into your menu rotation over the next month.

For Further Study: Study Psalm 103:5 in various translations and the original Hebrew for the various applications.

Genesis 1:29, Genesis 9:3, Psalm 78:24-25, Psalm 104:14, 27-28, Psalm 111:5, Psalm 145:15, Matthew 14:19, and Acts 14:17

_____

_____

_____

_____

_____

_____

_____

_____

_____

_____

_____

_____

_____

_____

Day 17: Be Bitter

A satisfied soul loathes the honeycomb, but to a hungry soul every bitter thing is sweet. Proverbs 27:7 (NKJV) ("Loathes" can be translated "tramples on.")

My Thoughts:

_____

_____

_____

What is with today's title? Of course, I do not mean that you need to be bitter in your emotions or in your spirit. I do mean, just like your grandmother may have told you, "Eat your vegetables."

Vegetables, especially green leafy ones, are classified as "bitter." According to this scripture, how do you best season your vegetables or any food? With hunger.

Let's look at today's scripture. "A satisfied soul loathes the honeycomb." Think back to a holiday feast when you came to the table hungry and everything tasted delicious. (Okay, maybe not the canned beets.) You ate each dish (except the beets). You enjoyed seconds. You stuffed in thirds. Lastly, you removed your belt to accommodate the pie and ice cream. After consuming a few days worth of food in an hour, even stretching out on the sofa did not relieve the pain. As you were contemplating changing into your sweat pants, your aunt brought out your favorite dessert. Ouch. Decisions. You knew you would be sick with even one bite. The taste would have been unexceptional and bland, so you "trampled" on your favorite, so to speak. You did not eat it (until later that night, of course). Strange that your beloved dessert did not appeal to you, yet an hour earlier, the spinach salad had tasted wonderful. Why?

This is science. Hunger heightens your taste buds' ability to taste and distinguish flavors and to pick up on the natural sugars in even "bitter" foods. However, with each bite your taste buds lose their sensitivity until cookies taste like cardboard.

When you wait until you are physically hungry to eat you increase the pleasure of food, even vegetables. Do you have trouble eating your vegetables or other "good things" which you listed yesterday? Perhaps you have snacked too much, and you are not coming to the table hungry. Maybe you are eating only because it is mealtime, according to the clock.

If you have trained your taste buds with excess sweets or junk food, anything not "super-sized" sweet will be bland to them. In this case, you may have to start retraining them to enjoy "bitter" foods with only a few bites of dark leafy greens, even when you are physically hungry.

Be careful to not go to the other extreme. Hunger should be pleasant. If you are light-headed, cannot concentrate, have a headache, or would be willing to tackle people to get to food, you have waited too long to eat. If the hunger is intermittent and you are saying, "I'm not sure if I am hungry," wait another 15-30 minutes to see if you become truly hungry. Pay attention to your hunger cues, so that you can "get hungry" but not "go hungry." We will discuss this concept further in *Day 19: Be Satisfied.*

Your Challenge:

Begin confessing "Today, I will wait until I am physically hungry to eat." Do not put food in your mouth until you have sensed physical hunger. If you are hungry and mealtime is not soon, snack enough to take the edge off of your hunger, but not enough to "ruin your dinner," as your mom would say.

For Further Study: Psalm 107:9, Matthew 5:6, and John 6:35

_____

_____

_____

_____

_____

_____

_____

_____

_____

_____

_____

_____

_____

_____

_____

_____

_____

Day 18: It's Time to Set the Table

She has prepared her food, she has mixed her wine; she has also set her table. Proverbs 9:2 (NASB)

My Thoughts:

_____

_____

_____

God wants you satisfied. We read that in Psalms 103:5 on *Day 16: It's a Good Thing*. Also, God "gives us richly all things to enjoy" (I Timothy 6:17, NKJV). "All things" includes food, right? God wants you to enjoy your meals!

Let's get the most pleasure we can from the food He has given to us. How?

1. **Wait:** Incorporate yesterday's lesson on waiting for gentle physical hunger.
2. **Experience the variety God made:** Your mouth can feel textures and temperatures. Your taste buds can distinguish between the varieties of apples. It is in food diversity that you receive the vast array of nutrients God designed for your body. A bowl of *just* lettuce – though lettuce is healthy – will not satisfy.
3. **Use your creativity in seasoning!** Boring meals will not satisfy. Plus, herbs and spices have numerous benefits beyond providing vitamins and

minerals. When I read Proverbs 31:14, I think of the exotic foods and spices likely served in the Proverbs 31 woman's home.

4. **Limit distractions:** *Where* you eat and *how* you eat can maximize meal enjoyment. Even delicious meals eaten in front of the TV or computer will not satisfy because you do not notice the texture, temperature, and taste. Also, when you eat while distracted, it is difficult to observe when you are no longer hungry (this is tomorrow's lesson).

5. **Plan and prepare your food:** Create anticipation for your meals by taking the time to make them. As we know from planning vacations and events, anticipation increases the pleasure. In most families today, we don't plan and cook our food. We grab something on the way home or open a can of soup. (I'm guilty of that, too. It decreases my enjoyment. I always experience more satisfaction when I prepare at least a portion of the meal.) Try these ideas and think of your own:

   - Take 15 minutes each week to review new recipes
   - Watch a cooking techniques video
   - Schedule one time each month to attempt a delicious, but challenging, dish. (Of course, recruit someone else to clean up the aftermath.)
   - Rotate theme nights. For example, play Italian music on pasta night or decorate for an indoor beach party when serving fish tacos.
   - Determine two or three nights each week when you will prioritize time to cook
   - On the weekend, plan your upcoming week's menu. Include in your menus both items you will purchase ready-made (bread, complicated side dishes, etc.) and food you will make yourself.
   - Cook basic ingredients in bulk. If three recipes for the week call for brown rice as the base, cook all of it at once to save time later.

- Pre-package your own snacks for the week at the same time: homemade trail mix, cut veggies with dip, boiled eggs, etc.
- Get your kids to help. This is a great way to teach them about food and nutrition. In fact, a friend and her daughter, prepared meals from scratch for a few months and they both lost weight "without trying."

6. **Set your table:** Create the atmosphere you want at your table, from the linens you use to the language you allow.

Your Challenge:

Ask the Holy Spirit to show you which of these ideas (or your own insights) He wants you to enjoy first. Experiment with it.

For Further Study: Proverbs 31:14, Ecclesiastes 2:24-25, John 12:2, 1 Timothy 6:17-19, and Revelation 19:9

Day 19: Be Satisfied

And they all ate and were satisfied, and they picked up what was left over of the broken pieces, seven large baskets full. Matthew 15:37 (NASB)

Now Boaz said to her at mealtime, 'Come here, and eat of the bread, and dip your piece of bread in the vinegar.' So she sat beside the reapers, and he passed parched grain to her; and she ate and was satisfied, and kept some back. Ruth 2:14 (NKJV)

My Thoughts:

_____

_____

_____

If you have ever dieted for more than a week or two, then you know that "I'm not satisfied" feeling. Once the excitement of a new diet wears off, the limited variety (cabbage soup, anyone?) or the limited amount (constant calorie counting), leaves your mouth or your stomach unsatisfied. That is not God's will, nor how He designed your body to self-regulate.

Does He mean you should stuff yourself with food? No. That is eating beyond satisfaction. The Bible has much to say about gluttony, too. When you eat when you are not hungry (which means you are still satisfied from the last meal), or when you eat past the point of satisfaction, you are overriding the regulation He built into your body. Anytime we overrule the system, we make it much more difficult next time to work with it. Notice in

Ruth 2:14 that Ruth did not leave the table hungry. Neither did she continue to eat once she fulfilled her hunger. "She ate and was satisfied, and kept some back."

If you consistently make yourself "go hungry" or, the other extreme, "eat when already satisfied," ask God to show you why. What is going on that you are overriding His plan? Fear of hunger, due to years of dieting? Fear of gaining weight? Boredom? Stress? The time on the clock? Or _____? Journal about your reasons either before or after you eat. After a couple of weeks, read your entries to look for any trends.

Acknowledge your discoveries, and then experiment with new ways of handling those thoughts, habits, or emotions.

Sometimes feeling "satisfied" or "no longer hungry" relates to *what* you ate. Ask yourself:

1. **What foods truly satisfy me?**

   _____

2. **What foods make me feel sluggish or hungry an hour later?**

   _____

Other times, feeling "satisfied" or "no longer hungry" is because of the amount of food or calories you ate. Pay attention to your body's signals for the answers to the following questions:

1. **What does my stomach and body feel like when I "eat and am satisfied?"**

   _____

2. **How do I know if I have under eaten or overeaten?**

   _____

Your Challenge:

Begin confessing, "I will learn what foods truly satisfy me; I will eat undistracted, and I'll stop eating when I am satisfied." As Proverbs 13:25 says, eat "to the satisfying." Don't go to either extreme. Get hungry, but don't go hungry. Do eat to the point of satisfaction and then stop, knowing that the next time you get hungry you will eat again.

A note to former dieters: Becoming re-attuned to the sensations of hunger and satisfaction will take time. You were born with the God-given ability to recognize hunger and fullness. Ask the Holy Spirit to help you re-learn to listen.

For Further Study: Deuteronomy 8:7-10, Deuteronomy 11:8-15, Psalm 107:9, Psalm 145:15-16, Proverbs 12:11, and Proverbs 13:25

_____

_____

_____

_____

_____

_____

_____

_____

_____

_____

_____

_____

_____

_____

_____

_____

Day 20: Be Joyful and Peaceful

Go, eat your bread with joy, And drink your wine with a merry heart;
For God has already accepted your works. Ecclesiastes 9:7 (NKJV)

Better is a dinner of herbs where love is, than a fatted calf with hatred. Proverbs 15:17 (NKJV)

My Thoughts:

_____

_____

_____

Let's go back to your high school biology class. (I know: moan, groan.) Remember the sympathetic and parasympathetic nervous systems? Only one of these systems can be dominant at a time. When you are agitated, excited, upset, in crisis, angry, or stressed the sympathetic nervous system is kicking into gear. This means that the parasympathetic system is not able to function well. You may recall that the parasympathetic system controls your digestive system.

Uh, oh. We have a situation. The exciting movie you are watching with dinner (re-read *Day 18: It's Time to Set the Table*), the argument you just had with your teenager, the mulling over what your coworker did, the worrying about whether someone accepts you, or the report that is due at work tomorrow each keep you from digesting your food well.

God knows what He is talking about when He instructs us to:

- Cast our cares on Him (1 Peter 5:7)
- Not worry (Matthew 6:25-34)
- Forgive and walk in love (1 Corinthians 13:4-7 and Ephesians 4:32)
- Think on things that are excellent and praiseworthy (Philippians 4:6-8)
- Receive the acceptance Jesus bought for us (Ecclesiastes 9:7; Ephesians 1:6 and 2:8; and Philippians 1:6).

Living in peace and joy is important anytime, but especially at mealtime! God wants you to be healthy. He knows that for you to digest your food well, which allows you to absorb the nutrients to "renew your youth," you need to be joyful and peaceful when you eat.

This also includes allowing God to be the emotional lift that you need. Many of us (especially those of us who were chronic dieters) have trained ourselves to dull (or distract) negative emotions through eating. When you are angry or sad or bored, before you open the pantry out of habit, tell God what you are feeling. Ask Him to show you how to process your emotions. God will give you strength to tolerate the discomfort until it naturally passes, which it often does. He will give you wisdom to change the thoughts causing the emotions. He will show you answers to stressful situations. God will heal your heartache.

Your Challenge:

When you pray before your meals today, also take a moment to cast your cares on God, to forgive someone, and to think about the good in your life. Then the food that He blessed can be a blessing to you.

For Further Study: Ecclesiastes 9:7; Matthew 6:25-34; 1 Corinthians 13:4-7; Ephesians 1:6, 2:8, and 4:32; Philippians 1:6 and 4:6-8; Philippians 1:61; and 1 Peter 5:7

_____

_____

_____

_____

_____

_____

_____

_____

_____

_____

_____

_____

_____

_____

_____

_____

_____

_____

Day 21: Drink up!

Jesus answered and said to her, "Everyone who drinks of this water will thirst again; but whoever drinks of the water that I will give him shall never thirst; but the water that I will give him will become in him a well of water springing up to eternal life. John 4:13-14 (NASB)

My Thoughts:

_____

_____

_____

I can relate to the woman of Samaria's physical thirst. When working in my garden in early June, with the heat index already in the mid-90's, quenching my thirst is paramount. After just 30 minutes of pulling weeds in the heat and humidity, I need to drink water. It's not a big deal for me to refresh myself though; I am blessed to have easy access to clean drinking water. I simply walk into my house and fill up my glass. Around the world, others have to travel half a mile or carry a heavy jar in the hot sun to a well like the Samaritan woman did. Many have to brave getting water from a river with crocodiles or deadly snakes.

Though acquiring water is vastly different for me than it was for the Samaritan woman, or is for others worldwide, we all do have one thing in common – we know water is essential to life. The amazing benefits of water in my body motivate me to drink it consistently. Let's talk about them.

90

- Everything that happens in your body's cells goes on in a base of water
- "Water naturally suppresses the appetite and helps the body metabolize stored fat. Studies have shown that a decrease in water intake causes fat deposits to increase, while increasing water intake can actually reduce fat deposits."
- "Water...is the medium for transporting molecules in and out of cells"
- "Water lubricates joints and acts as a shock absorber"
- "Water is contained in the eye as well as in the spinal cord"

No wonder we feel great when we drink enough water, and we have lower energy when we don't! Water makes up 55-60% of your body; therefore, it is delivered to "vital organs" first when you are slightly dehydrated.[iv] If you notice your skin is a little drier or more wrinkled than usual, or – how shall I say this delicately? – if you deal with constipation, then you probably need to drink more water.

How much water should you drink each day? That amount is individual. I have listed a few websites in the appendix to help you determine that answer for your body. Even without the calculations though, you can use the principle taught in Psalm 103:5 about how good things renew your youth.

As you read today's scriptures, notice that when people were thirsty God did not bless them with milk or wine (or soda or ...). He blessed them with *water*. For many people, simply replacing the man-made drinks with what God made for the body will take care of their water needs. Try swapping out sodas, pre-mixed flavor packets, and energy drinks for plain or naturally flavored water (lemon slices, cucumber slices, herb infusions, etc.). The appendix includes a fun website for fruit and herb infusions.

Your Challenge:

If you drink man-made drinks, begin switching some of them for water. Evaluate your body's signals and your energy level. How does your body tell you that it needs more water? Remember: God loves you and what He has created for you is best.

Pray for those around the world who have to risk their lives to get water. In fact, be part of the solution to help assess and provide a community's water needs, whether they be a new well, rainwater collection and storage, water purification, or sanitation training.

Check out www.africaoasisproject.org to find out more. You can donate through Cornerstone Church Nashville, 726 West Old Hickory Boulevard, Madison, TN 37115, or www.cornerstonenashville.org. Designate "Africa Oasis Project." One hundred percent of your donation will go to help supply clean water to the people of Africa.

For Further Study: Exodus 17:1-6, 1 Kings 17, Joshua 15:18-20, Judges 15:18-20, Psalm 107:35, and Revelation 7:16-17

_____

_____

_____

_____

_____

_____

_____

_____

_____

_____

_____

_____

_____

_____

_____

_____

Week 4

What Else Does the Bible Say about Health?

Day 22: From A(wake) to Zzz

Unless the LORD builds the house, they labor in vain who build it; unless the LORD guards the city, the watchman keeps awake in vain. It is vain for you to rise up early, to retire late, to eat the bread of painful labors; for He gives to His beloved even in his sleep. Psalm 127: 1-2 (NASB)

Unless the LORD builds the house, they labor in vain who build it; unless the LORD guards the city, the watchman stays awake in vain. It is vain for you to rise up early, to sit up late, to eat the bread of sorrows; for so He gives His beloved sleep. Psalm 127:1-2 (NKJV)

My Thoughts:

_____

_____

_____

An infant needs 14-15 hours of sleep. An adult needs around seven to eight hours of sleep. Contrary to popular opinion, sleep is not a luxury. We need sleep as much as air, water and food. Sleep not only makes life more enjoyable, it is critical to our health and success in life.

Here's how getting enough sleep will help you:

- Better concentration
- Greater memory and planning skills
- Improved weight management

- Creative problem solving, even while you sleep
- Toxins removed from brain and body
- Muscles and organs healed
- Slower aging of skin and brain
- Decreased risk of Alzheimer's Disease

Extreme sleep deprivation also is a safety issue. According to Dr. Charles Czeisler, faculty member at the Harvard Medical School, "We now know that 24 hours without sleep, or a week of sleeping four or five hours a night, induces an impairment equivalent to a blood alcohol level of 0.1%. We would never say, 'This person is a great worker – he's drunk all the time,' yet we continue to celebrate people who sacrifice sleep for work."[v]

So, what can you do to help get your zzz's?

1. **Accept that sleep is important to your success.** Athletes and top professionals are now prioritizing their sleep schedules as much as other healthy lifestyle habits.
2. **Know that God will take care of the issues which keep you up late and cause you to worry.** Compare the two translations of our scripture today. He wants to bless you *with* sleep and He wants to bring blessings to you *while* you sleep. He cannot do that if you are trusting in yourself to solve problems at midnight. God stays awake to solve them for you.
3. **Follow the basics of sleep hygiene.**
   - Do not look at a TV, a computer, or a blue light device (smartphone, tablet, etc.) before bedtime. (Experiment with the time frame you need. I require at least an hour without screen light before falling asleep.)
   - Get as much natural light during the day as possible. Work near a window or walk outside at lunchtime.
   - Exercise regularly
   - Add light-blocking window shades and set a cooler temperature in your bedroom

- Do not drink alcohol or eat a heavy meal before bed
- Set a regular sleep schedule of when to go to bed and when to wake, not varying by more than an hour on the weekend
- Meditate on a calming or encouraging Bible verse before you go to sleep. Read a story in the Old Testament.
- If you wake up in the middle of the night, know that that is often normal. Relax and read your Bible. When you get sleepy again, go back to bed.

If you follow these three steps, yet consistently have trouble with sleeping, seek professional help. Your health and success are worth it!

Your Challenge:

Find and read scriptures that comfort you before you go to sleep. When my mind or emotions struggle, I find these passages helpful: Isaiah 41:10; Psalm 37, 91, and 119; Philippians 4:4-9; and Hebrews 4.

For Further Study: Psalm 4:8, Psalm 121:4, and Proverbs 3:24

_____

_____

_____

_____

_____

_____

_____

_____

_____

_____

_____

_____

_____

_____

_____

_____

_____

100

Day 23: Don't be Mocked

Wine is a mocker, strong drink a brawler, and whoever is intoxicated by it is not wise. Proverbs 20:1 (NASB)

For the heavy drinker and the glutton will come to poverty, and drowsiness will clothe one with rags. Proverbs 23:21 (NASB)

My Thoughts:

_____

_____

_____

The consumption of alcohol is a controversial subject in the church. Denominations and individuals have a wide range of views. Regardless of your personal convictions, one fact all Christians can agree upon is that alcohol has a strong physiological health impact that we cannot ignore.

The Bible instructs us that wine will mock and that drinking until intoxicated is not wise. Unfortunately, crossing the line to intoxication is way too easy. This is one reason to seriously pray and seek wise counsel concerning drinking. Alcohol affects your body and your life. I encourage you to research its impact on families, crime, industry and accidents. The statistics change yearly, but are always shocking.

Today let's focus on the basic well-documented health impact. As Dr. Dick Couey discusses in *Happiness Is Being a Physically Fit Christian*, alcohol increases your risk of ulcers. It inhibits your ability to use iron to make hemoglobin, the molecule which carries oxygen in your blood. Consistent alcohol use decreases your immune function. Moderate drinking increases the development of arteriosclerosis.[vi] Alcohol also increases a woman's risk of breast cancer.

According to Jared Tanner, Ph.D. in clinical psychology, "Alcohol easily crosses the blood brain barrier, which serves to protect the brain from harmful substances...and [alcohol] directly affects the neurotransmitters and receptors of neurons. At high enough concentrations (or over time) alcohol can weaken the blood brain barrier."[vii] Alcohol damages your cognitive ability and can allow toxins into your brain.

Your Challenge:

If you do not drink, don't think of yourself as being "more holy" than those who do. (That's a 2 Corinthians 10:12 study.) But do know that you are making a positive choice for yourself. If you do drink, consider how alcohol affects your body, and if you are being a good steward of your body. If you drink heavily, please seek help.

Further Study: Leviticus 10:9-10, Proverbs 23:29-31, Proverbs 31:4-6, Isaiah 28:1 and 7, Ephesians 5:18, and 1 Timothy 3:2-3

_____

_____

_____

_____

_____

_____

_____

_____

_____

_____

_____

_____

_____

_____

_____

_____

Day 24: The No-Stress Zone

Casting the whole of your care [all your anxieties, all your worries, all your concerns, once and for all] on Him, for He cares for you affectionately and cares about you watchfully. 1 Peter 5:7 (AMP)

Rejoice in the Lord always; again I will say, rejoice! Let your gentle spirit be known to all men. The Lord is near. Be anxious for nothing, but in everything by prayer and supplication with thanksgiving let your requests be made known to God. And the peace of God, which surpasses all comprehension, will guard your hearts and your minds in Christ Jesus. Philippians 4:4-7 (NASB)

My Thoughts:

_____

_____

_____

Stress is a major factor in most lifestyle diseases. According to The American Institute of Stress, 77% of people regularly suffer physical problems caused by stress. Stress costs American industry more than $300 *billion* annually, through health care and missed work.[viii]

We were designed for Eden. We were made for bliss. We were not designed for a fallen world or all it contains. God did not originally create our bodies and minds to handle grief, arguments, troubles, or tragedy.

104

Unfortunately, we live in a world of tribulation. In fact, in John 16:33 Jesus even goes so far as to tell us we will have pressure and problems. Our physical, mental, and emotional systems were not formed to handle the hardships that Jesus says we will experience. Knowing this may leave us feeling helpless and frustrated. It's like reading a "whodunit" mystery, only to discover someone tore out the last chapter, and we are left without the answer.

Take heart! God wouldn't leave us in an unresolved situation. He provides many solutions in the Bible.

1. **Get God's Perspective.** Much (most?) stress relates to what you think about a situation *more* than the situation itself. "People are disturbed not by a thing, but by their perception of a thing" – Epictetus. To counter our concerns, Philippians 4:8 tells you to think on the good stuff. (More on that in *Day 25: Take Captive*.)
2. **Chill out.** Meditate on 1 Peter 5:7. Tell yourself, "God's got this!" You do what you can do in the natural and believe God will do what only He can do in the supernatural. Refuse to worry.
3. **Say no.** Some sources of stress are self-inflicted. If you commit your time to activities God hasn't instructed you to do, you end up with more promises and projects than you have hours in the day to complete. That feels stressful just thinking about it. Proverbs 31:16a says, "She considers a [new] field before she buys *or* accepts it [expanding prudently and not courting neglect of her present duties by assuming other duties]" (AMP).
4. **Set boundaries.** It is pretty stressful when you let your boundaries get crossed! Learn to control how your time, emotional strength, and every facet of your life is shared or protected. Check out the appendix for great books on setting healthy boundaries.
5. **Take care of yourself.** A little time invested exercising, reading and praying during quiet time alone (Mark 1:35), doing something pleasurable

(Psalm 16:11), and focusing on good nutrition will recharge your body and emotions. Don't neglect self-care, even when you are busy.
6. **Forgive and be forgiven.** Receive God's forgiveness, forgive others, and forgive yourself. Let go of bitterness, guilt and shame.
7. **Rely on the supernatural strength of God, through your spirit.** As stated earlier, your body, mind, and emotions were not originally formed to deal with a fallen world. But read Ephesians 3:16 and 6:10-17. Your spirit can be guided and strengthened by your Creator to make you mighty!

Your Challenge:

Pray that God will show you one area or action you can change to better manage stress. Your thoughts. Your commitments. Self-care. Boundaries. Casting your cares on Him. Forgiveness. Once He reveals it, take a step forward.

For Further Study: Psalm 27:1 and 3; Psalm 37:3-5; Psalm 139:23; Proverbs 3:5-6; Proverbs 12:25; Isaiah 41:10; Isaiah 55:8-9; Jeremiah 33:3; Matthew 6:25-34; Mark 6:46; Philippians 4:4-6 and 19; and Hebrews 4:3

_____

_____

_____

_____

_____

_____

_____

_____

_____

_____

_____

_____

_____

_____

_____

_____

Day 25: Take Captive

For the weapons of our warfare are not carnal but mighty in God for pulling down strongholds, casting down arguments and every high thing that exalts itself against the knowledge of God, bringing every thought into captivity to the obedience of Christ. 2 Corinthians 10:4-5 (NKJV)

Finally, brethren, whatever is true, whatever is honorable, whatever is right, whatever is pure, whatever is lovely, whatever is of good repute, if there is any excellence and if anything worthy of praise, dwell on these things. Philippians 4:8 (NASB)

Pleasant words are as a honeycomb, sweet to the mind and healing to the body. Proverbs 16:24 (AMP)

Death and life are in the power of the tongue, And those who love it will eat its fruit. Proverbs 18:21 (NKJV)

My Thoughts:

_____

_____

Related to yesterday's lesson on stress management is the power of what we think. Should we take captive immoral thoughts? Yes. But we also must corral negative and worrisome thoughts.

Your thoughts are so powerful they will impact your health and even the length of your life! Multiple research studies compare individuals of similar health who hold varied beliefs about their health status. Those who view their health as poor die at an earlier age than those who view their health as good, even though their actual health is the same. Charles Capps, in his book, *God's Creative Power ® for Healing* comments on some of these studies. He concluded that individuals with a self-image of poor health, "even though they may be in good health, they seem to live out the reality of the image they have of themselves even unto death."[ix]

What you focus on will grow strong in your life. Like rain, sun, and soil are to plants, your thoughts are to your life. Picture what you want in your life and then picture your thoughts raining on and nourishing that desire. Ask yourself, "What's feeding my thoughts?" TV and the Internet? Books? The Bible? The devil? You are responsible to fill your mind with God's Word so that your thoughts bring peace, joy, and health into your life.

Focus only on thoughts that line up with the Word. If you think, "I don't know if I can cook healthy," instead tell yourself, "God is giving me the resources I need to cook nutritious and enjoyable foods." If you think, "I don't like to walk," instead confess, "I enjoy taking a break each day and seeing God's creation while I walk." If you think, "I'm worried about my health," instead say God's Word about your health. Whatever the harmful thought, replace it with what you *want* to see grow in your life.

Scripture teaches us to be proactive in our thought life. Don't wait for a destructive thought to show up and say, "Hmmm ... now what is something good to think in place of this negative thought?" Do like King David did: train your mind *daily* by meditating on God's Word and His works. Then, if a negative thought tries to come in, you can recognize it and replace it with the truth of Scripture.

As you are proactive about your thought life, invest some time each day to "dream big." Exciting dreams give you energy. Get involved in a dream bigger than yourself.

Never, ever limit what you think God can do. Read
Ephesians 3:20; you can't out-dream God!

Your Challenge:

Keep a sheet of paper with you today. When you
recognize a negative thought, write down what you want
to think instead. Start reading your "replacement
thoughts" every day.

For Further Study: Genesis 24:63, Joshua 1:8, Psalm 1:2, Psalm 4:4, Psalm 77:12, Psalm 143:5, Proverbs 3:1-8, Jeremiah 29:11, Romans 8:6, 1 Corinthians 2:16, 1 Corinthians 13:5, Ephesians 3:20

_____

_____

_____

_____

_____

_____

_____

_____

_____

_____

_____

_____

_____

_____

_____

_____

Day 26: Relationships

Not forsaking our own assembling together, as is the habit of some, but encouraging one another; and all the more as you see the day drawing near. Hebrews 10:25 (NASB)

Day by day continuing with one mind in the temple, and breaking bread from house to house, they were taking their meals together with gladness and sincerity of heart. Acts 2:46 (NASB)

My Thoughts:

_____

_____

_____

Even though Adam was in relationship with God, God said it was not good that Adam be alone. He remedied this by creating another human being, Eve. God made us for relationships. Having healthy ones positively impacts our physical health.

In the book *Emotional Longevity: What Really Determines How Long You Live*, Norman B. Anderson, Ph.D., relates several research studies which show the benefits of a strong social network. In one study with more than 2,000 participants, "a number of social relationships were measured, including marital status, church attendance, and participation in volunteer
112

activities. Women with smaller social networks had a mortality rate nearly double that of those high in social ties ... men low in social ties died at two to three times the rate of men with strong social connections."

Other studies referenced showed the following:

- "Relationships predict heart-disease deaths ... [and] heart attack recovery"
- "Relationships predict against the common cold"
- "Relationships predict birth outcomes"
- "Relationships predict hypertension...atherosclerosis...[and] stress-hormone levels"
- "Relationships affect immune-system status"[x]

One way to decrease stress (see *Day 24: The No-Stress Zone*) is to be in healthy relationships that are mutually beneficial. Our stress decreases when we know we have people we can lean on when we're not strong. (Is that tune going through your head now, too?) "Lean on" means others offer us emotional and practical support, whether we're in a crisis or simply need help moving furniture. A network of friends also provides mental support: others help you think through issues.

Growing up, I rode to and from school every day with my mother. (She was my high school English teacher.) We were each other's "sounding boards." Each morning and afternoon, we'd toss dilemmas and ideas off one another as a means of emotional and mental support. I need that still today as an adult. You need that. We need people who support us and to whom we provide support.

If you struggle to form healthy relationships or if you have trouble with boundaries in relationships, read the books suggested in the appendix.

Your Challenge:

Think of one relationship you would like to improve this week. What you can do to improve it? Take that first step today.

For Further Study: Genesis 2:18, 1 Samuel 18:1-4, Job 42:10, Proverbs 17:17, Ecclesiastes 4:9-12, John 11:1-44, John 15:13, Acts 27:3, Romans 12:18

_____

_____

_____

_____

_____

_____

_____

_____

_____

_____

_____

_____

_____

_____

_____

_____

Day 27: Divine Healing

Who Himself bore our sins in His own body on the tree, that we, having died to sins, might live for righteousness – by whose stripes you were healed. 1 Peter 2:24 (NKJV)

He sent His Word and healed them, and delivered them from their destructions. Psalm 107:20 (NKJV)

My Thoughts:

_____

_____

_____

Here are three questions I ask in my *Go Forward: Eat, Move, and Enjoy Life God's Way* workshops:

1. Does divine forgiveness mean we can live in sin? (Read 1 Peter 2:24.)
2. Then does our right to divine healing mean we can live unhealthy?
3. Does living healthy negate the need for Jesus' stripes?

The answer is no to all three questions. First, Jesus' crucifixion and wounds free us from the curse of the law (Galatians 3:10-13), which includes sickness (Deuteronomy 28:58-61). Second, we still live in a fallen

116

world with a real devil who hates us and wants to destroy us (John 10:10). We need both the sacrifice of Jesus and healthy living.

As we have seen over the past 26 days, God cares about our health habits. Even in Numbers and Leviticus, we read God's instructions to the Israelites on everything from sanitation to preventing the spread of infections. However, God does not just provide us guidance on health practices to lower our risk of disease. He also gives us access to divine healing through the stripes of Jesus. He has done His part. Our part is to live healthy, seek medical attention when necessary, and build our faith for divine health.

The English word for "saved" or "salvation" is translated from the Greek word "sozo." Sozo also means "deliver, protect, heal, preserve, and make whole." I'm believing that on my way to heaven, God will grant me all of that down here!

If you have questions about divine health or healing, please invest time studying God's Word and books which explore this topic in depth. It can be a challenging subject. Above all, know that God loves you and wants you to be healthy.

Your Challenge:

Do what you need to do in the natural and the spiritual to be a steward of your body.

1. Find a great book on divine healing and read it. (Suggested readings are listed in the appendix.)
2. Every time you steward your body in the natural, whether going for a walk, watching a sunset to relax or eating your vegetables, also think or speak a scripture on health.

For Further Study: Psalm 103:3, Jeremiah 30:17, Matthew 9:18-10:8, Matthew 20:34, Mark 1:29-31, Acts 5:16, 1 Corinthians 12:28, James 5:14-15, and 3 John 2

_____

_____

_____

_____

_____

_____

_____

_____

_____

_____

_____

_____

_____

_____

_____

_____

Day 28: You're a Human, Being Transformed

But we all, with unveiled face, beholding as in a mirror the glory of the Lord, are being transformed into the same image from glory to glory, just as from the Lord, the Spirit. 2 Corinthians 3:18 (NASB)

And do not be conformed to this world, but be transformed by the renewing of your mind, that you may prove what is that good and acceptable and perfect will of God. Romans 12:2 (NKJV)

My Thoughts:

_____

_____

_____

As much as we would all like to automatically, without effort, have everything we want happen all at once (by yesterday), we are human. We must choose what is most important to focus on now, and then as that habit becomes easier, decide what is next.

Here is an experiment that helped me to understand "transforming over time." I did this years ago at the beach and challenge you to do the same. Choose a day to wake up before the dawn to watch a sunrise from night until day. The sun does not suddenly pop up every morning. It transforms the sky over time. A sunrise is a process of over an hour. The sky melds from a deep black into a sheer gray. The gray transforms into a hint of color. Almost leisurely the pinks and oranges begin to appear and then become vibrant, wrapping from east to west. On it goes until the sun is above the horizon.

Incorporating an overall healthy lifestyle, for lasting change – not a fad diet or frenzied exercise program for two weeks before a vacation or class reunion – is a process. It happens in stages. Perhaps when you started this devotional, you began to drink a little more water. Maybe you added a 15 minute walk at lunch. Now, you might realize you need to increase your water intake again or start to strength train in the evening instead of watching TV (or at least *while* watching TV).

Here's the encouraging thing: as long as the sky keeps changing, slowly, we know the sun will cross the horizon and begin a new day. Keep watching your life's "sky." If it is a little lighter this week than last week, you are being transformed. Your "sky" – your habits – probably show a little more color now than 28 days ago. Keep working and believing. Your sun will come up.

Your Challenge:

We're back at the beginning. Ask God "What is the next step on my journey?"

What is next for you?

- Re-study a day or week that challenged you
- Develop an accountability relationship
- Mark your calendar to re-study this devotional guide in three months, to see how far you have come
- Find a friend to go through this study with you again
- Add another vegetable serving a day
- Walk another mile each day

120

- Call someone to mend a relationship
- Go to bed earlier each night
- Start to journal
- Read something funny every day
- Get an annual physical
- Schedule a session with a certified trainer or registered dietician
- Read a book on divine healing

For Further Study: Philippians 1:6

_____

_____

_____

_____

_____

_____

_____

_____

_____

_____

_____

_____

_____

_____

_____

_____

_____

_____

The Day After: Go Forward

Thank you for walking part of your journey of health with me. Like you, I will keep moving forward to improve my health. We will not always live "perfect" in our health habits this side of heaven. Do not let that discourage you; let it take the pressure off of you as you learn and grow. I'd like to share a moment of my journey with you that I pray will inspire you.

I was praying about an unhealthy nutrition practice I'd had since the age of nine. I felt scared to move to the next level. The new habit felt foreign to me, as do all new habits. It was emotionally painful for me to let go of the old and start the new.

Each evening I like to read a chapter or two in the Bible before going to sleep. One night, as I lay there considering the new habit, I "just happened" to read Exodus 14. (Don't you love God's "just happened" moments?) In this chapter, the Israelites stand trapped at the edge of the Red Sea, with the Egyptian army pursuing them. They think they have been led to the wilderness to die; out of desperate fear, they declare they prefer the familiar bondage in Egypt.

I could relate. My old pattern was familiar. I did not know what to expect out of a new habit. I was uncomfortable, even fearful. "If I change this, what may happen? What if I 'die' emotionally out there in this new way of living? I have never done this. What if I fail?" I wanted the comfortable road of the way I knew instead of the uncomfortable path to a new habit. (A new habit *is* an uncomfortable path. Two rocky steps forward, one stumbled step back. Though it will get easier over time, a change of thinking or acting does not happen instantly or effortlessly.)

From Exodus 14 the answer vaulted off the page into my spirit: a conviction, a directive, and a loving mandate. What God said to the Israelites in Exodus 14:15, He said to me. "Go forward." Ignore the irrational fear. Trust Him. "Go forward." I knew I needed a visual reminder to keep my mind focused on the new way of living (see *Day Two: Changing Habits*). The next morning I found a tiny gold bracelet in my jewelry box I decided to wear all day, every day. This piece of jewelry serves as my constant cue to push ahead in my health journey. While I have stumbled more than one step back at times, overall I am further in my journey. In the end, that is what matters.

You can, and will, continue further on your path, too.

"Go forward."

Appendix

Recommended Reading and Resources

Aging

Anderson, Norman, and P. Elizabeth Anderson. 2003. *Emotional Longevity: What Really Determines How Long You Live.* New York: Penguin Books.

Divine Healing

Bosworth, F.F. 1973. *Christ the Healer.* Grand Rapids, Michigan: Fleming H. Revell.

Hagin, Kenneth E. 1969. *Healing Belongs to Us.* Tulsa, OK: Faith Library Publications.

Hagin, Kenneth E. 1979. *Seven Things You Should Know about Divine Healing.* Tulsa, OK: Faith Library Publications.

Hayes, Norvel. 1986. *How to Live and Not Die.* Tulsa, OK: Harrison House.

Eating Disorders Help

American Psychological Association: http://locator.apa.org/

National Institutes of Mental Health: www.nimh.nih.gov/health/find-help/index.shtml

Exercise

American Council on Exercise: www.acefitness.org/acefit/locate-trainer/

Healthy Eating and Why Traditional Diets Do Not Work

Antonello, Jean. 1996. *Breaking Out of Food Jail: How to Free Yourself from Diets and Problem Eating Once and for All.* New York: Touchstone.

Fain, Jean. 2011. *The Self-Compassion Diet: A Step-by-Step Program to Lose Weight with Loving-Kindness.* Boulder, CO: Sounds True.

Guiliano, Mireille. 2007. *French Women Don't Get Fat: The Secret of Eating for Pleasure.* New York: Vintage Books.

Hansen, Vikki, and Shawn Goodman. 1997. *The 7 Secrets of Slim People.* New York: HarperPaperbacks.

Schwartz, Bob. 1996. *Diets Don't Work: Stop Dieting Become Naturally Thin Live a Diet-Free Life.* Houston, TX: Breakthru.

Somov, Pavel. 2008. *Eating the Moment: 141 Mindful Practices to Overcome Overeating One Meal at a Time.* Oakland, CA: New Harbinger.

Tribole, Evelyn, and Elyse Resch. 2003. *Intuitive Eating: A Revolutionary Program that Works.* New York: St. Martin's Press.

Relationships

Cloud, Henry, and John Townsend. 1992. *Boundaries.* Grand Rapids, Michigan: Zondervan.

Cloud, Henry, and John Townsend. 2005. *How to Have that Difficult Conversation You've Been Avoiding.* Grand Rapids, Michigan: Zondervan.

Eggerichs, Emerson. 2004. *Love and Respect.* Brentwood, TN: Integrity.

Katherine, Anne. 2000. *Where to Draw the Line: How to Set Healthy Boundaries Every Day.* New York: Fireside.

O'Neil, Mike, and Charles Newbold. 1994. *Boundary Power: How I Treat You, How I Let You Treat Me, How I Treat Myself.* Nashville, TN: Sonlight.

Water

http://nutrition.about.com/library/blwatercalculator.htm (Note: This website link ends in "htm" vs "html")

http://www.csgnetwork.com/humanh2owater.html

http://wellnessmama.com/3607/herb-fruit-infused-water/

About the Author

Sheri Traxler, M.Ed., holds her Master's Degree in Health Promotion, is an ACE Certified Personal Trainer, an AASDN Nutrition Specialist, and a Certified Intuitive Eating Counselor.

Sheri's work experience includes children's recreation programming, sports management, teaching Corporate Wellness courses at Belmont University, and cardiac rehabilitation. She worked at the Vanderbilt Dayani Center for Health and Wellness for 12 years as an exercise physiologist, membership director and Weight Management instructor. After leaving Vanderbilt, Sheri began health coaching, personal training, and teaching wellness workshops through her business, ViREO *Life*. She has been personal training clients for over 20 years.

Sheri is one of those "fortunate folks" who knew from childhood what she wanted to do: help people stay well. Her passion for exercise and healthy eating took a not-so-healthy turn at a young age. "I went on my first diet to lose two pounds at nine years of age." Dieting and disordered eating led to symptoms of anorexia by middle school. "I enjoyed exercise and how it gave me energy and made me feel strong. But because I worried about my weight, I would constantly count calories and fret about food. In my mid-twenties I read the books *Breaking Out of Food Jail* and *Diets Don't Work*. These books began a journey of learning about normal eating, while staying aware of the good nutrition information I had acquired in my college courses."

Her personal understanding of food struggles allows Sheri to help people who want to stop yo-yo dieting and learn to eat intuitively and healthy. These concepts are related as eating intuitively includes listening to the "health signals" from your body.

"I have always loved exercise and how it gives you energy and health to do everything else you want to do in life.

Whether hiking, running on the beach, weight training, or stretching, I enjoy moving. But, I understand folks who don't have that inclination. It is fun for me to help people find a style of movement that fits their lifestyle, from taking the stairs to training for races."

Sheri's mission is to create opportunities for individuals to find their unique path and abundantly live at their potential – physically, mentally and emotionally – based on spiritual truth.

To contact Sheri and for information about how she can help you, visit www.thevireolife.com

About ViREO *Life*

"Vireo" is Latin for "I flourish. I thrive. I am strong and active." Living a ViREO Life is to be, do, and enjoy all that God created for you. ViREO Life exists so that you can flourish, thrive, and be strong and active in *your* life.

Notes

[i] Hayford, Jack and Dick Mills (1991). *The Spirit Filled Life Bible*. Word Wealth p. 1802. Nashville, TN: HarperCollins Christian.

[ii] "Thin Cats." Graph. *Forbes*. January 20, 2014. p. 20.

[iii] Constitution of the World Health Organization. July 22, 1946. Basic Documents. Forty-fifth edition supplement. October 2006, accessed October 29,2015,http://www.who.int/governance/eb/who_constitution_en.pdf. Used with permission.

[iv] Pentz, J., G. Salgueiro, and S. Hauber. (2008). *Nutrition for Professionals*. pp. 16-17. West Roxbury, MA: LMA Publishing. Used with permission.

[v] Czeisler, Charles and Bronwyn Fryer. (October 2006). "Sleep Deficit: The Performance Killer, A Conversation with Harvard Medical School Professor Charles A. Czeisler," *Harvard Business Review*. Boston, MA: Harvard Business Publishing. Used with permission.

[vi] Couey, Dick. (1985). *Happiness Is Being a Physically Fit Christian*, pp. 163-165. Nashville, TN: B&H Publishing. Used with permission.

[vii] Tanner, Jared. September 12, 2008. "Physiological Effects of Alcohol Consumption," *Brain Blogger*. http://brainblogger.com/2008/09/12/physiological-effects-of-alcohol-consumption/. Used with permission.

[viii] . American Institute of Health. "2014 Stress Statistics." http://www.stress.org/daily-life/

[ix] Capps, Charles. (1991). *God's Creative Power ® for Healing*, p. 6. England, AR: Capps Publishing. Reprinted with permission from Charles Capps Ministries, Inc. November 2015

[x] Anderson, Norman and P. Elizabeth Anderson. (2003). *Emotional Longevity: What Really Determines How Long You Live*, pp. 117-135. New York: Penguin Books. Used with permission.

Made in the USA
Columbia, SC
07 April 2019